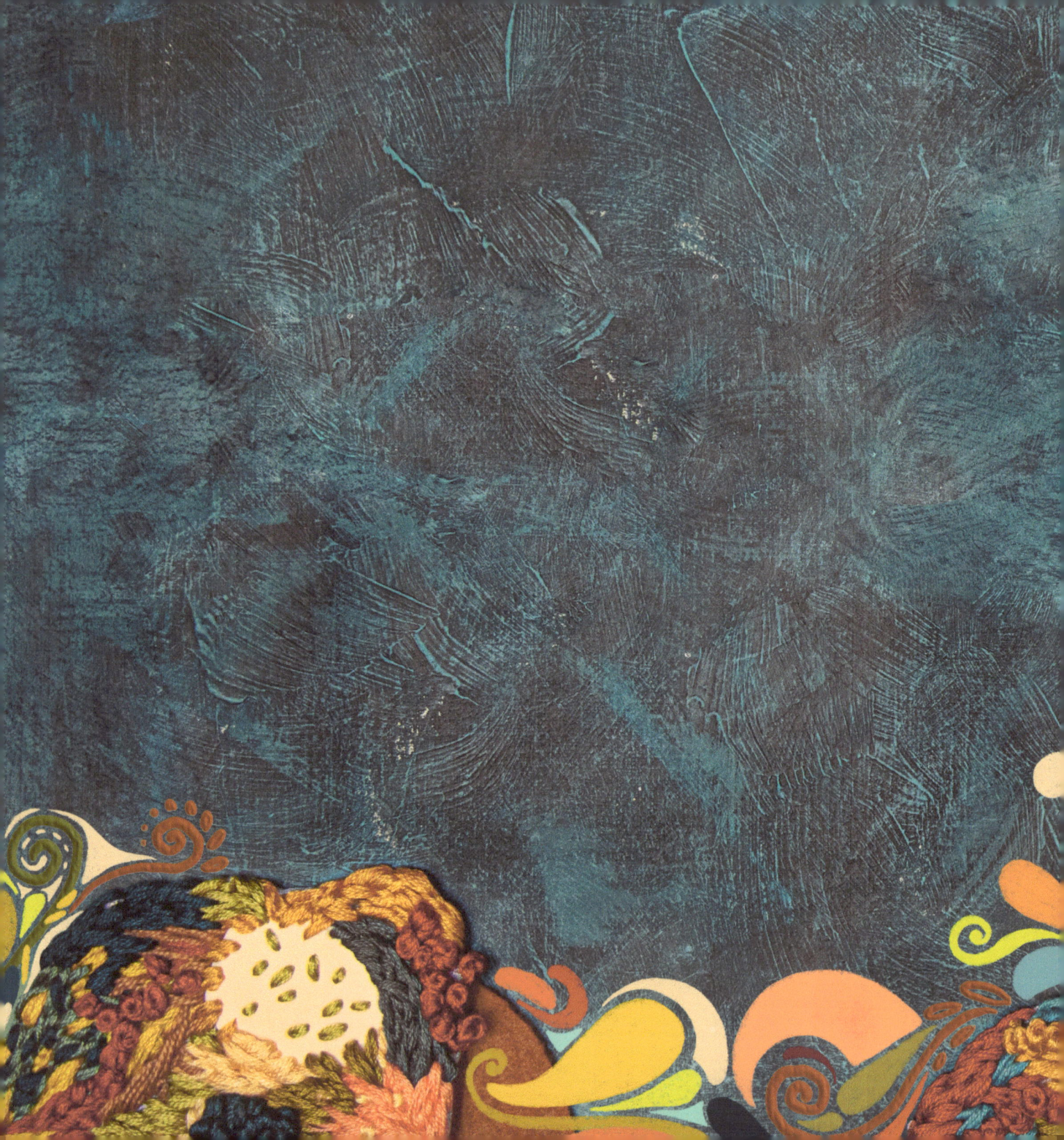

This book is dedicated to all who
observe the world with curiosity and
a willingness to try something new.

Hush Little Mind by Saskia Soliz

Published by Pinpoint+ Skills Lab, LLC

www.pinpointskillslab.com

Cover by Lola Svetlova

Thank you to Dr. Ehren Werntz and content creators

Isbn: 979-8-218-11919-5 (Paperback)

Isbn: 978-1-0880-0233-9 (Ebook)

Printed in USA

First Edition

HUSH LITTLE MIND

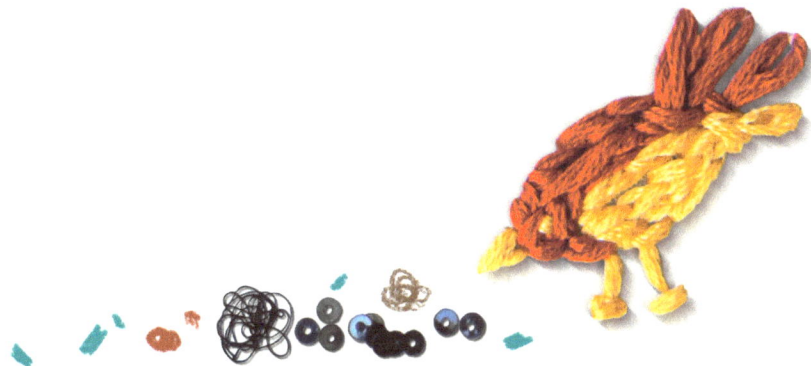

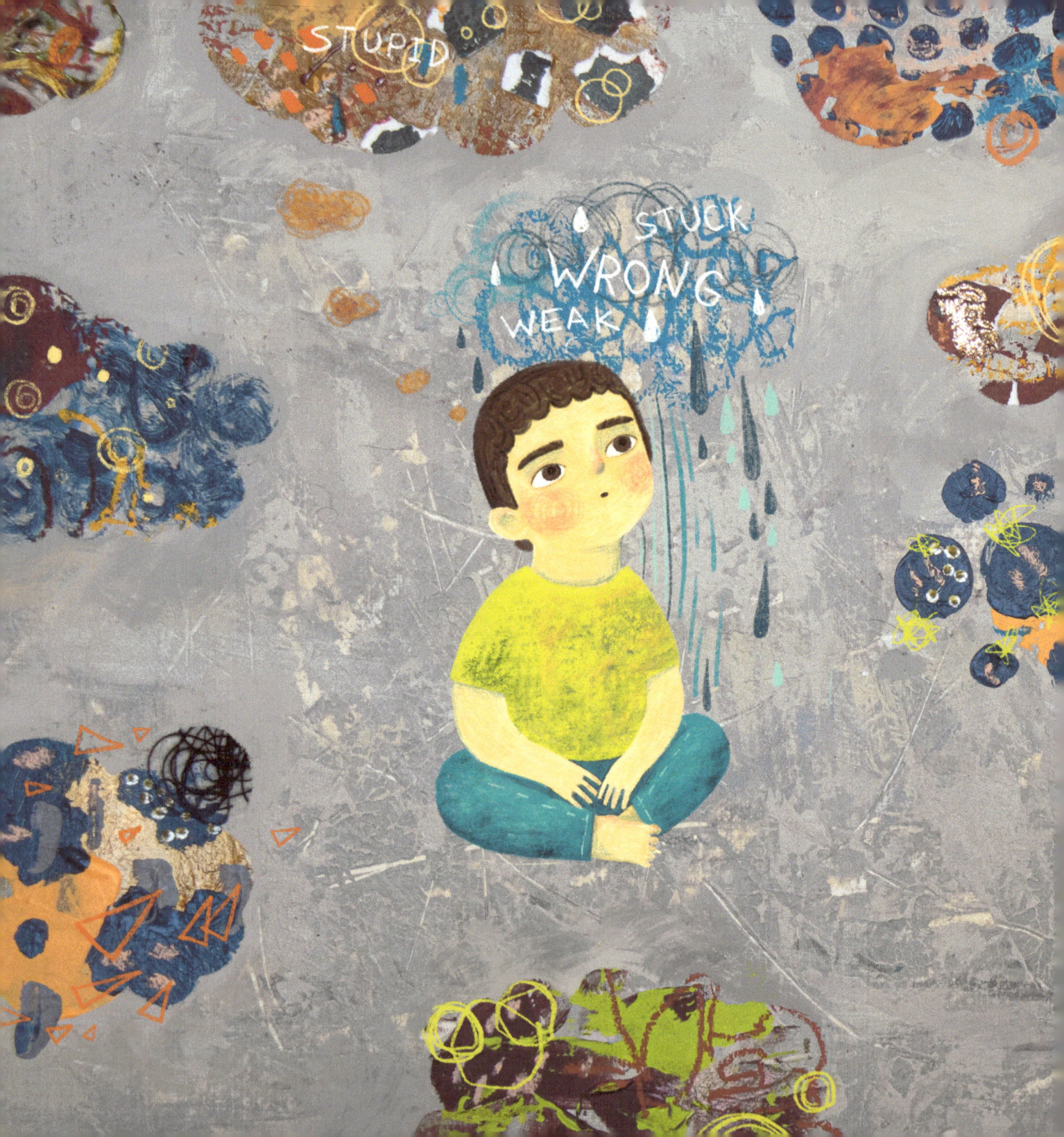

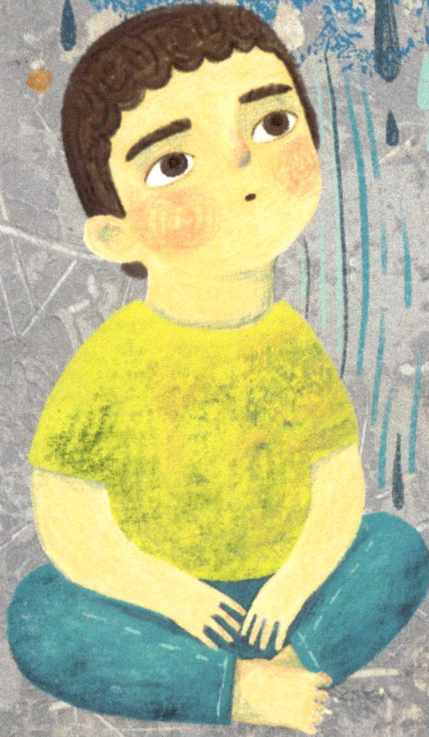

FAILURE

I KNOW YOU HAVE

A LOT TO SAY,

BUT SOME OF YOUR WORDS

ARE NOT HELPFUL TODAY.

WEIRD

YOU SEE,
I'VE FOUND MY DIRECTION,
MY NORTH STAR.

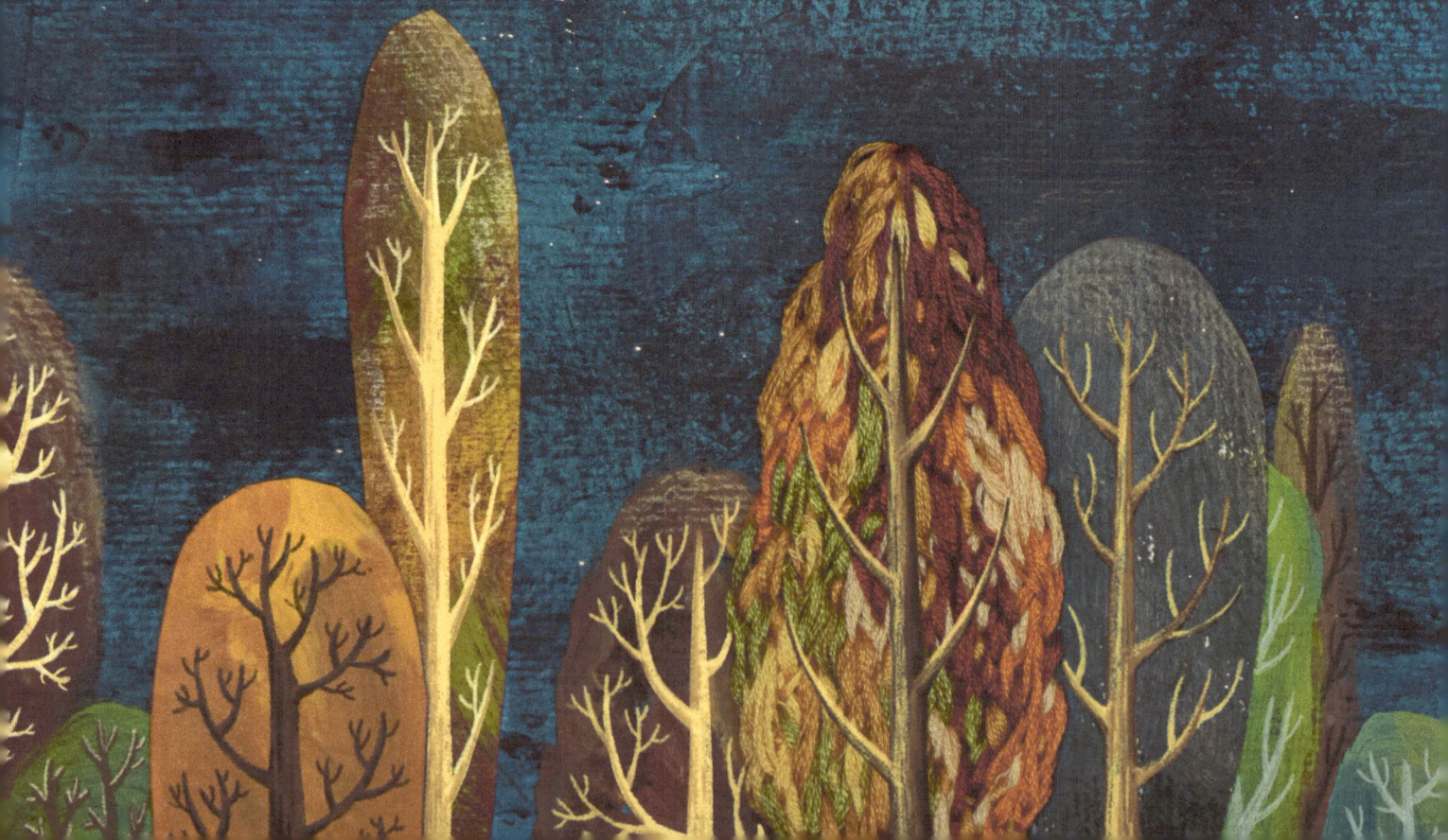

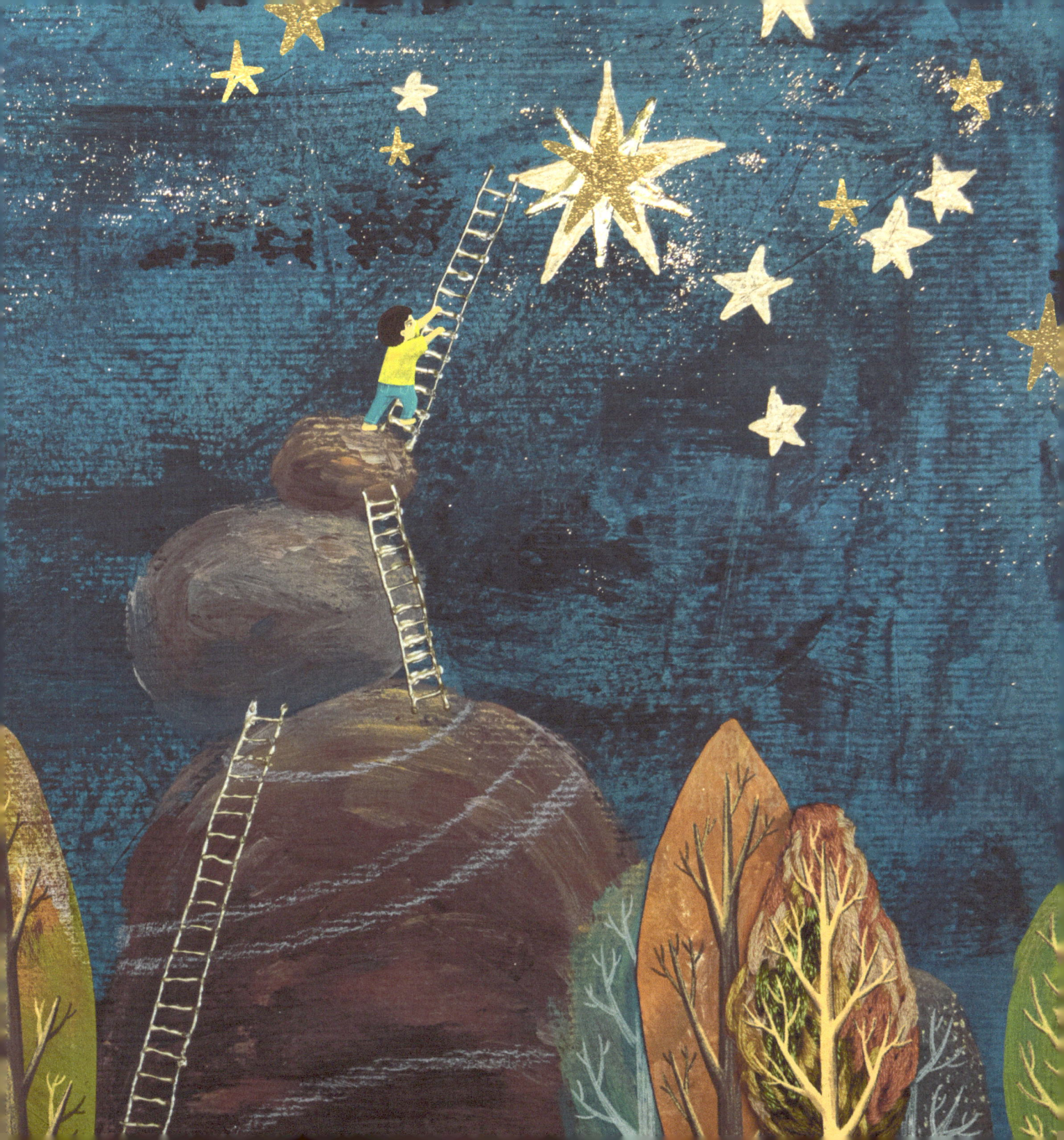

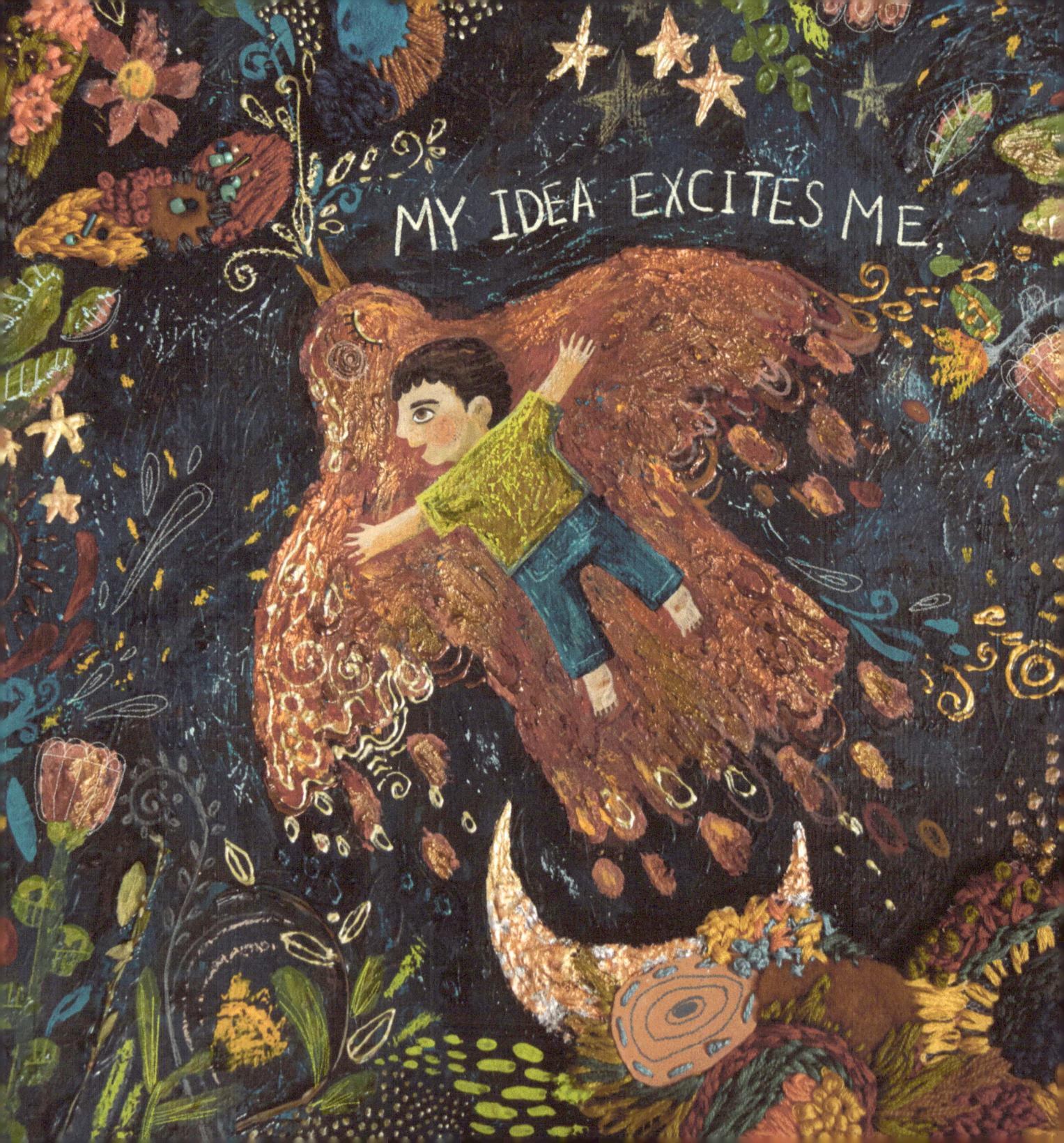

MY IDEA EXCITES ME,

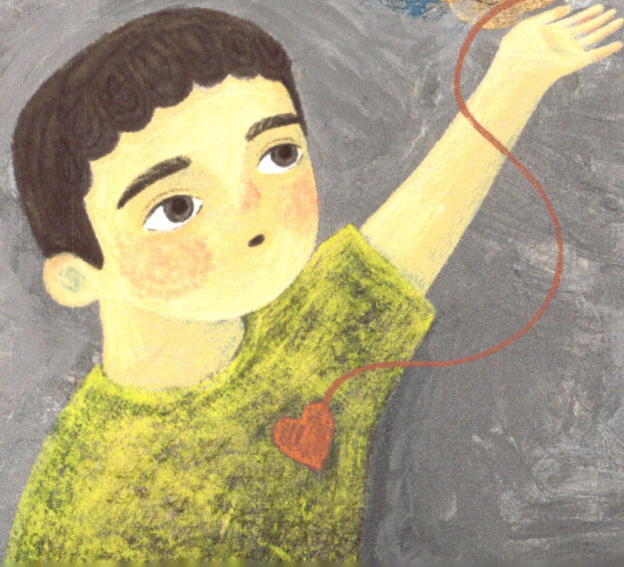

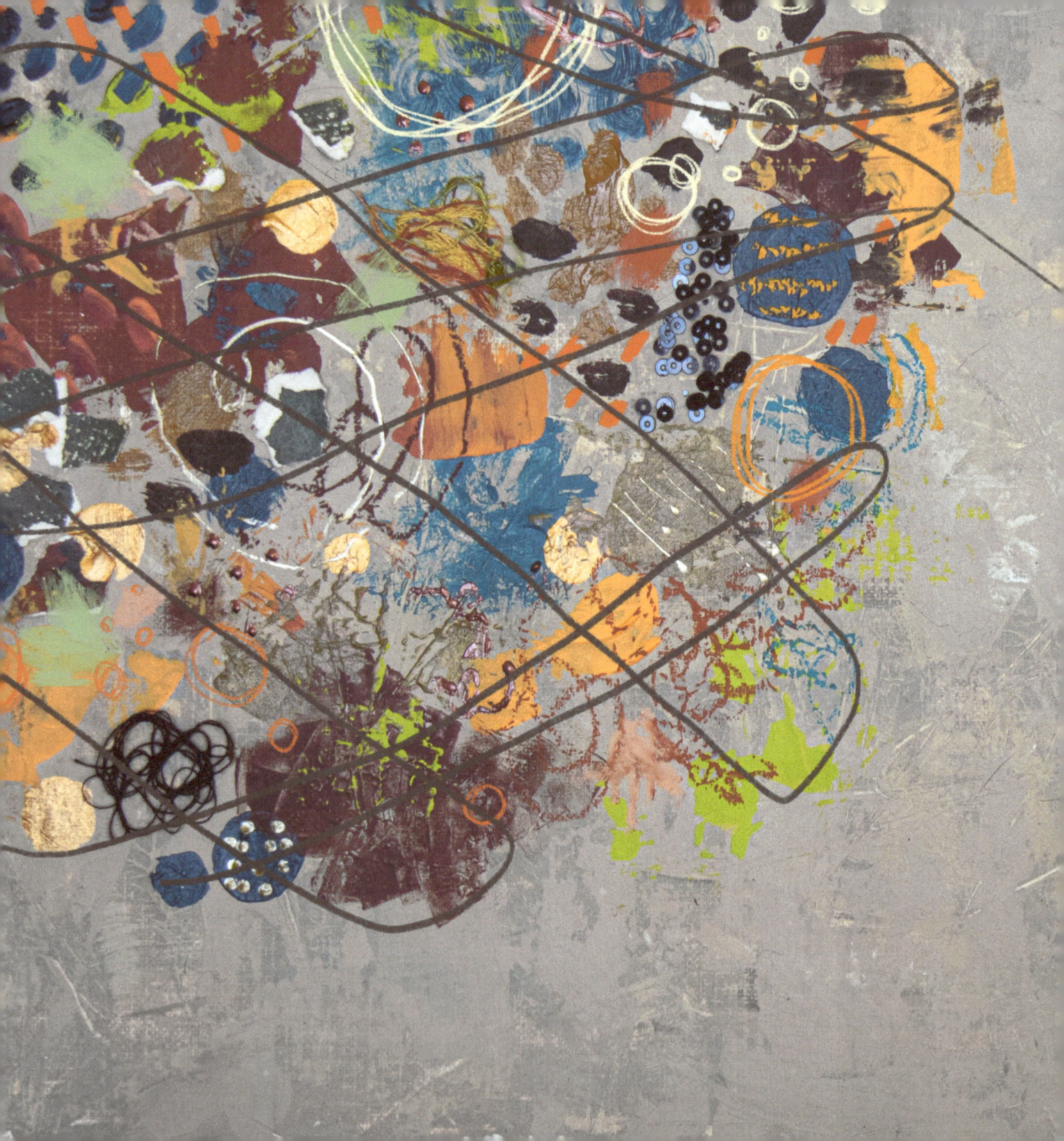

WHEN I HOLD
WHAT YOU SAY
JUST A LITTLE
TOO TIGHT...

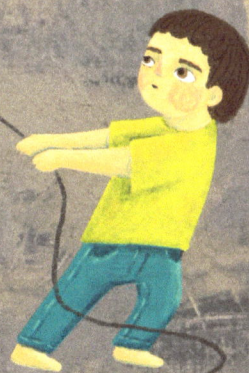

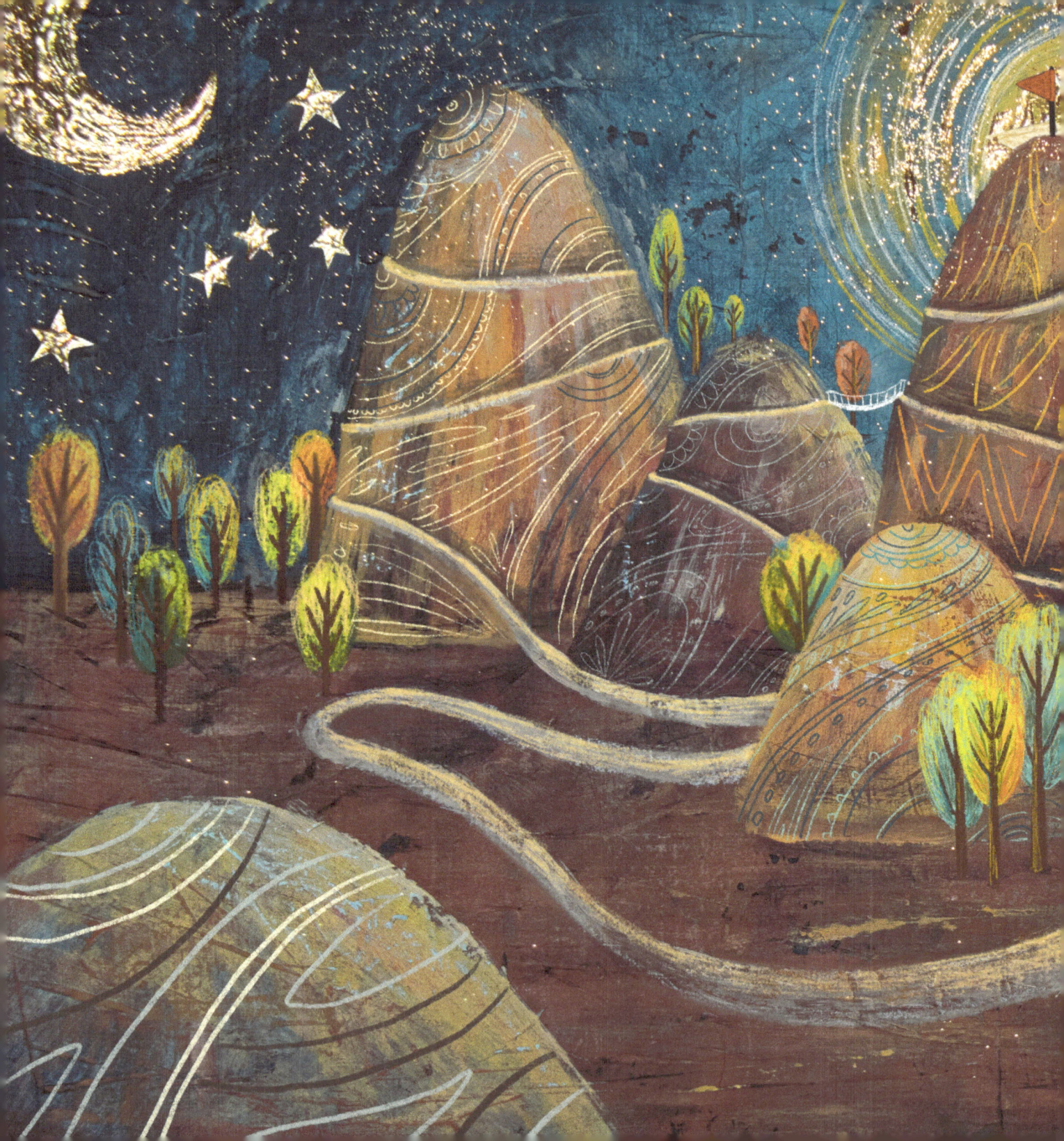

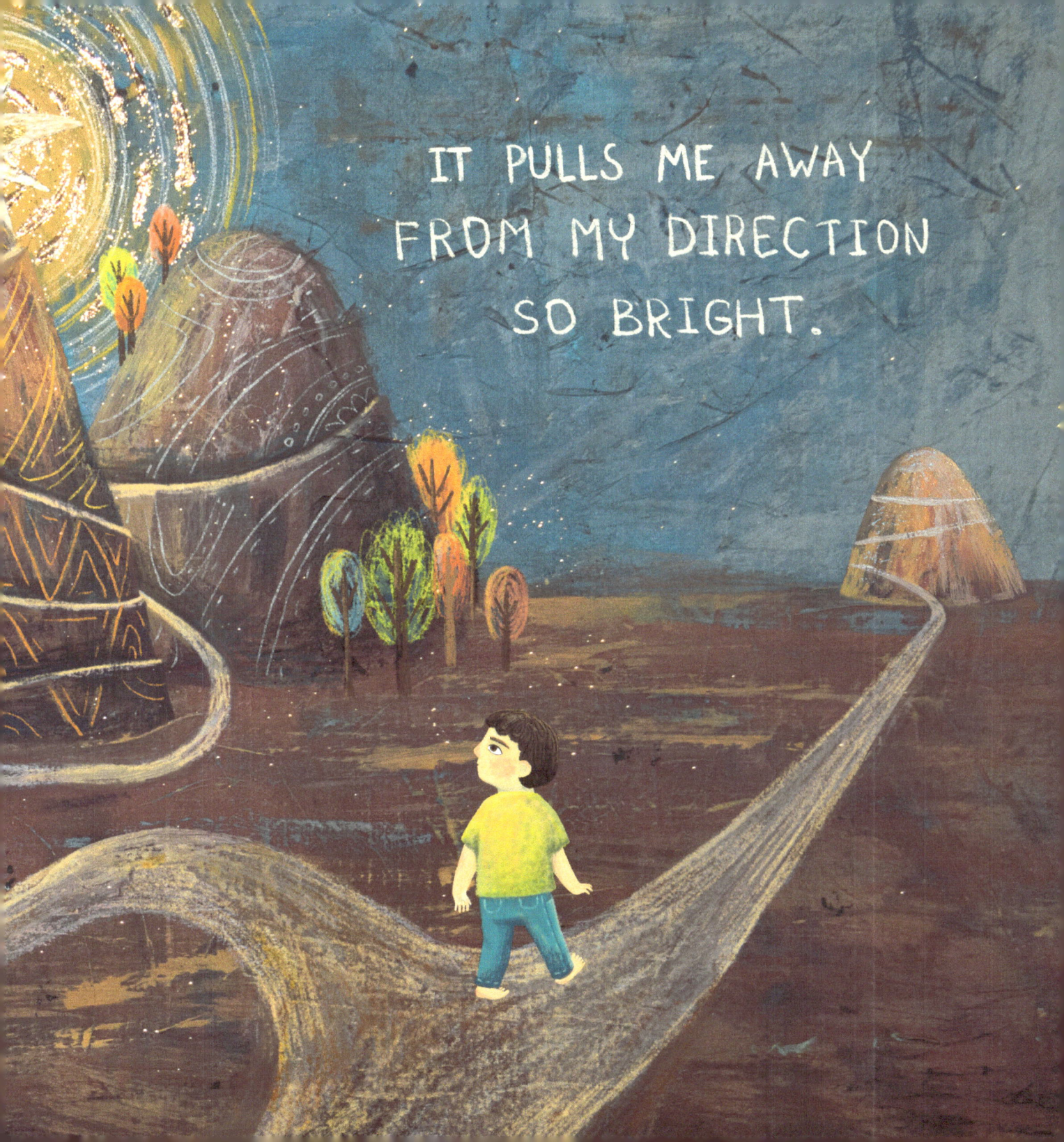

IT PULLS ME AWAY
FROM MY DIRECTION
SO BRIGHT.

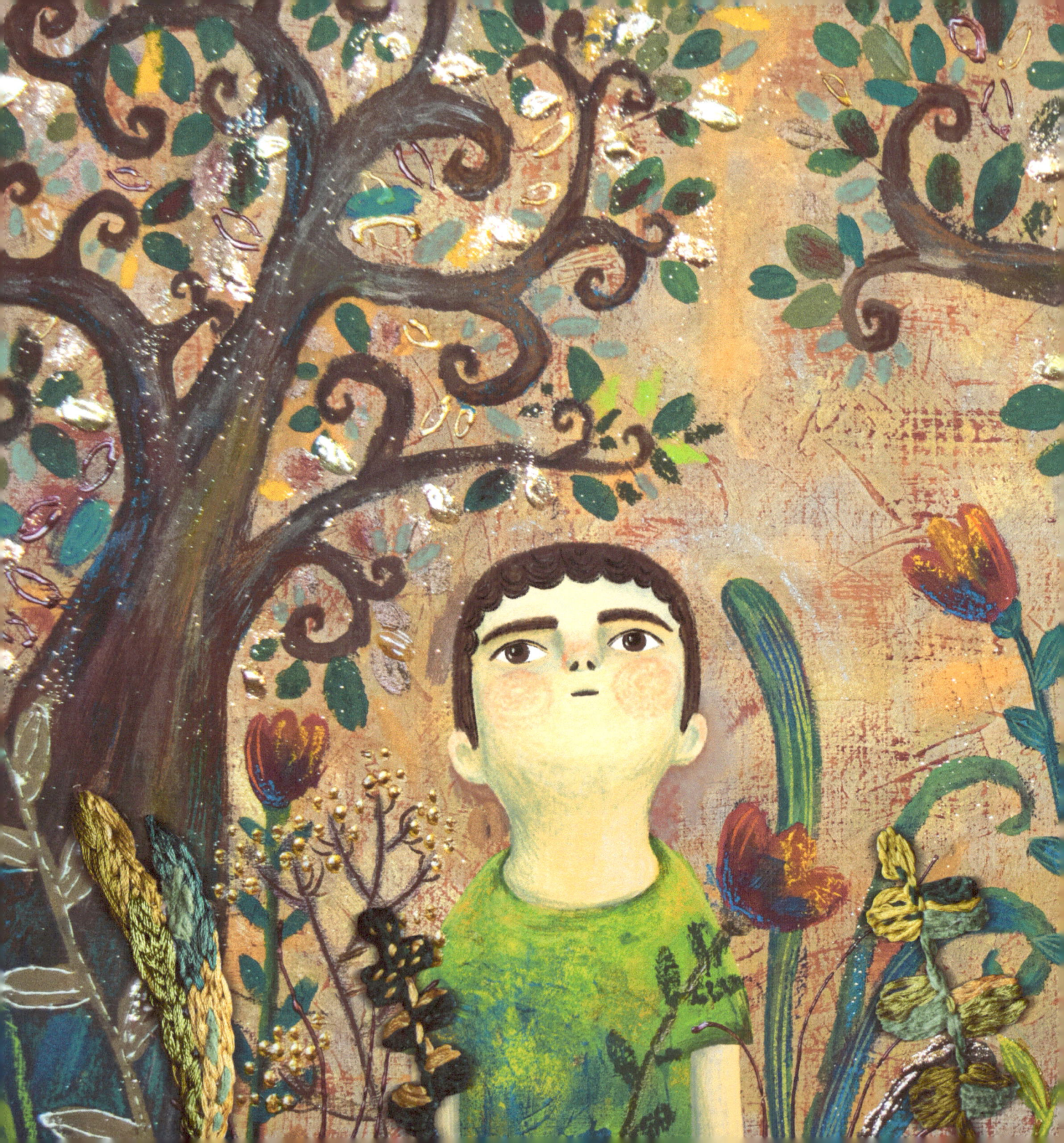

YES, THERE ARE THINGS
I CANNOT CHANGE,
BUT I AM MORE THAN THAT,
SO AGAIN I'LL SAY...

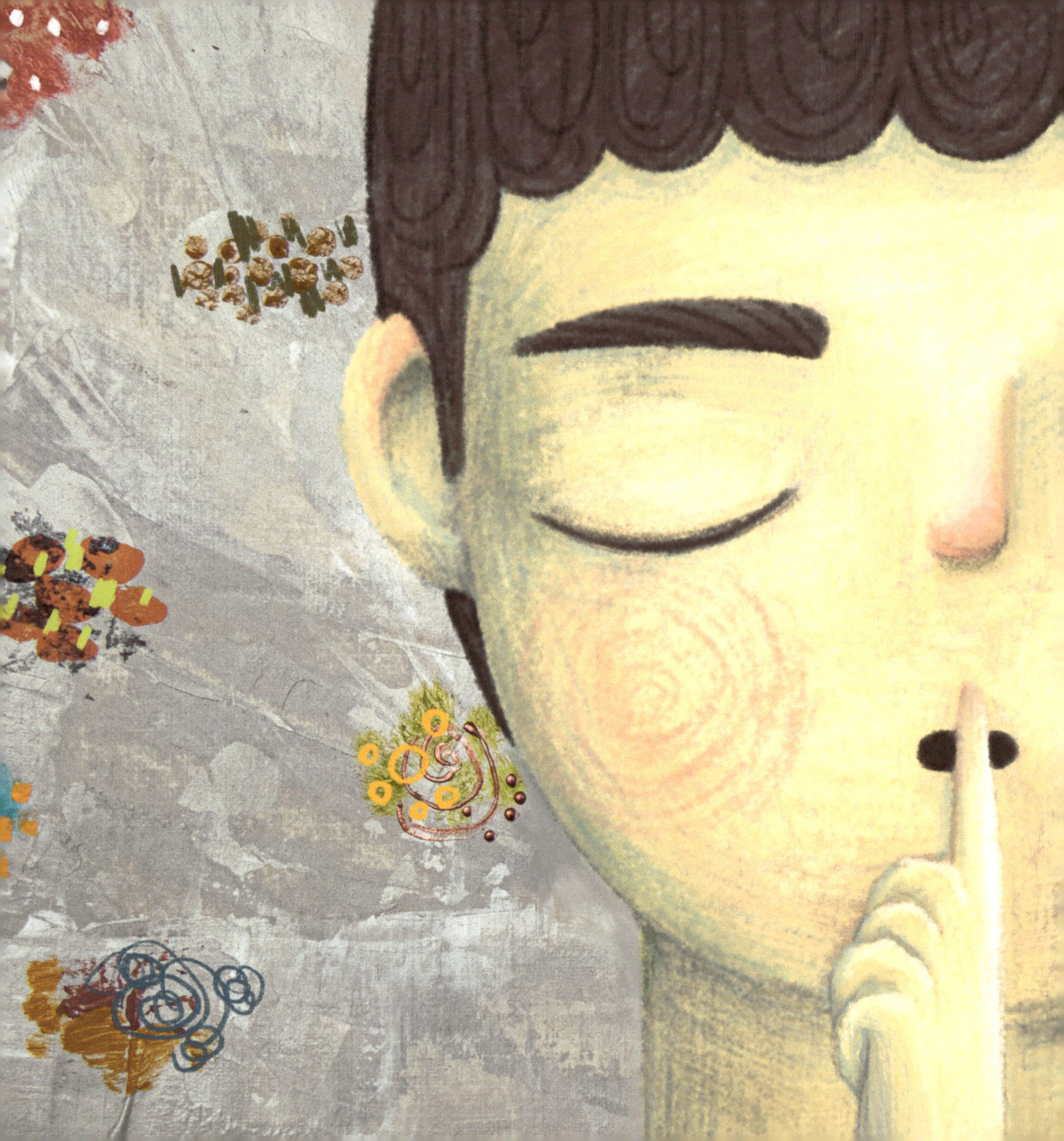

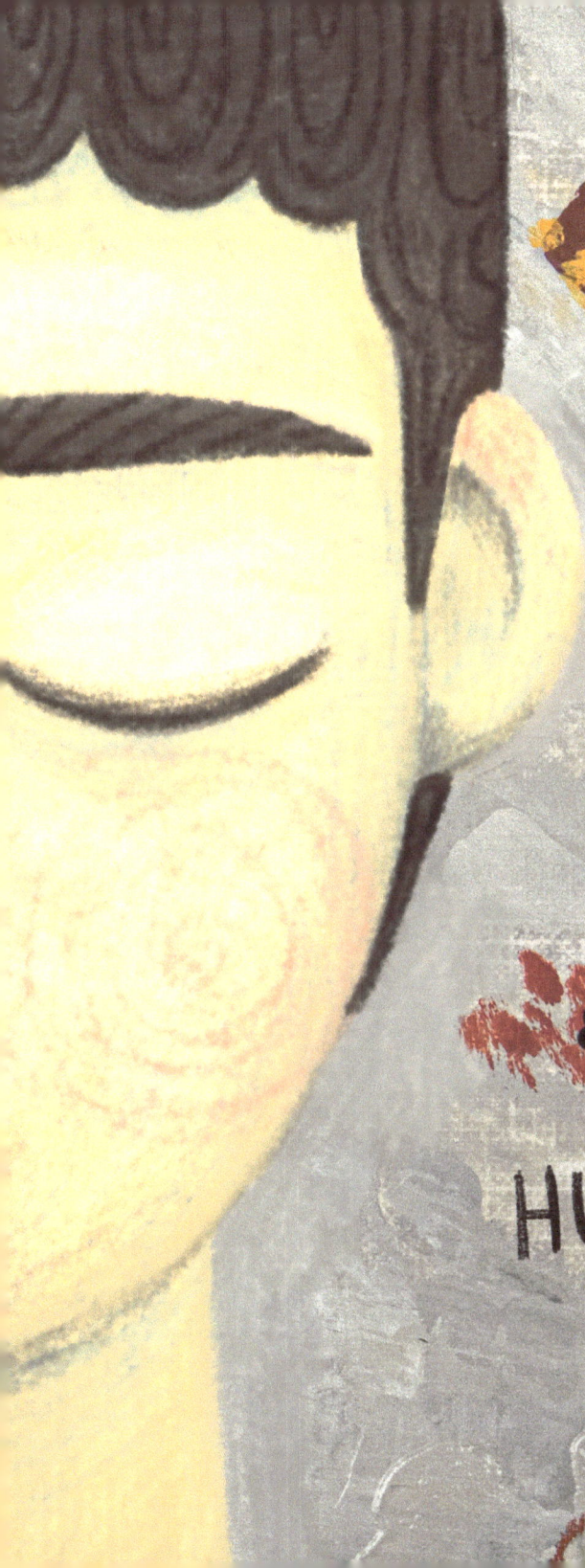

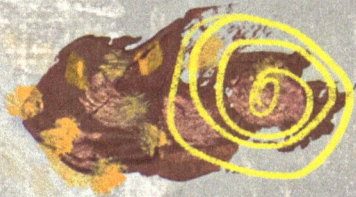

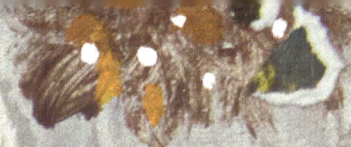

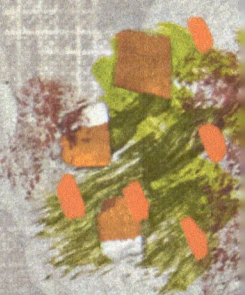

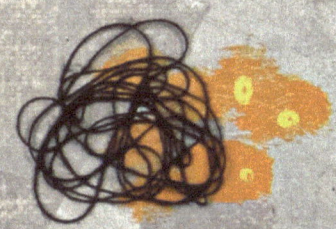

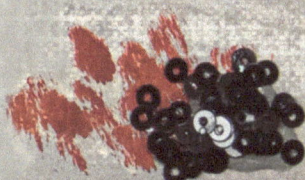

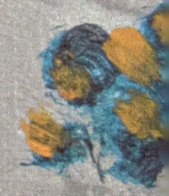

HUSH, LITTLE MIND.
REST TODAY.

I HAVE A FUN GAME,
WOULD YOU LIKE TO PLAY?

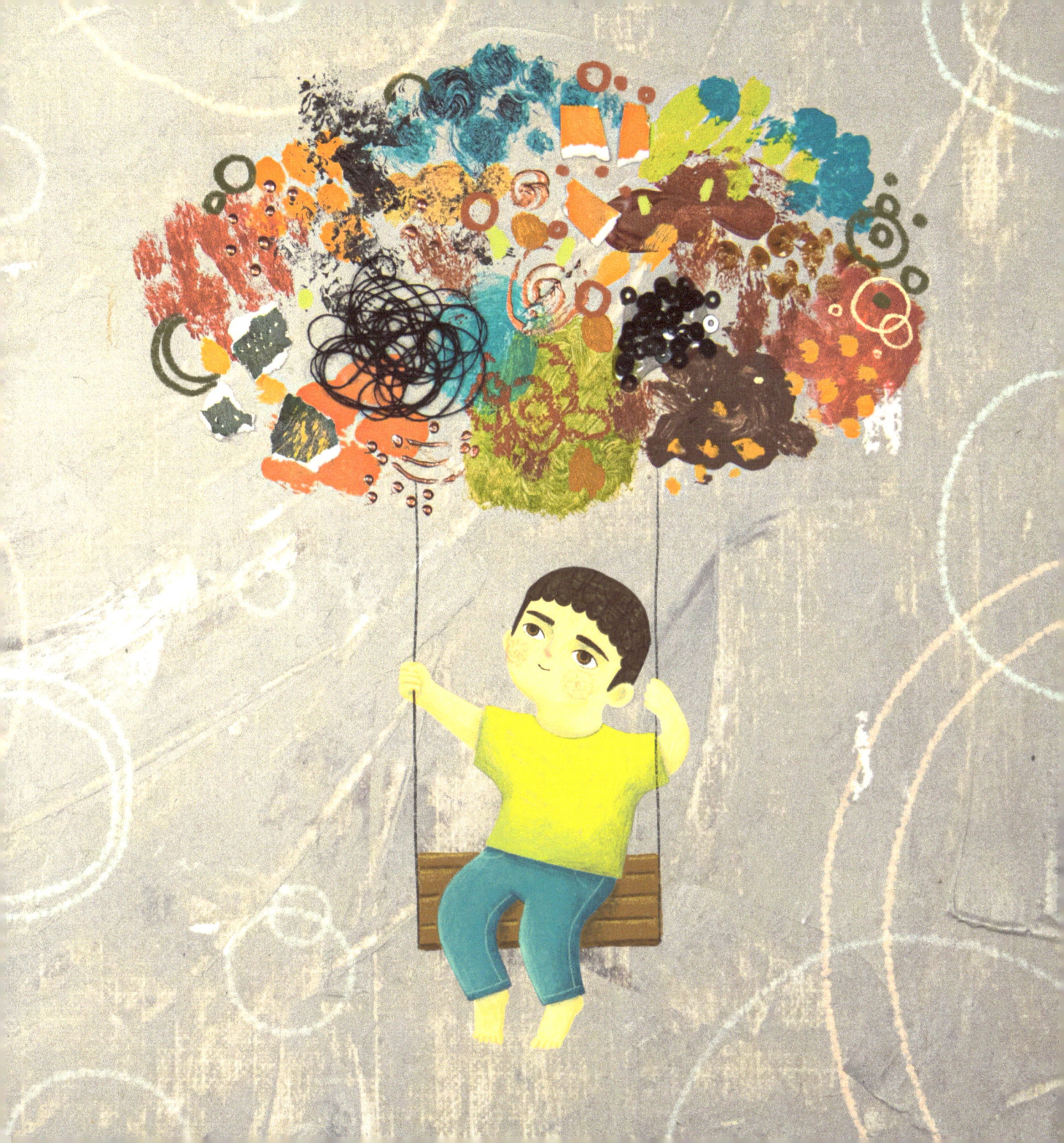

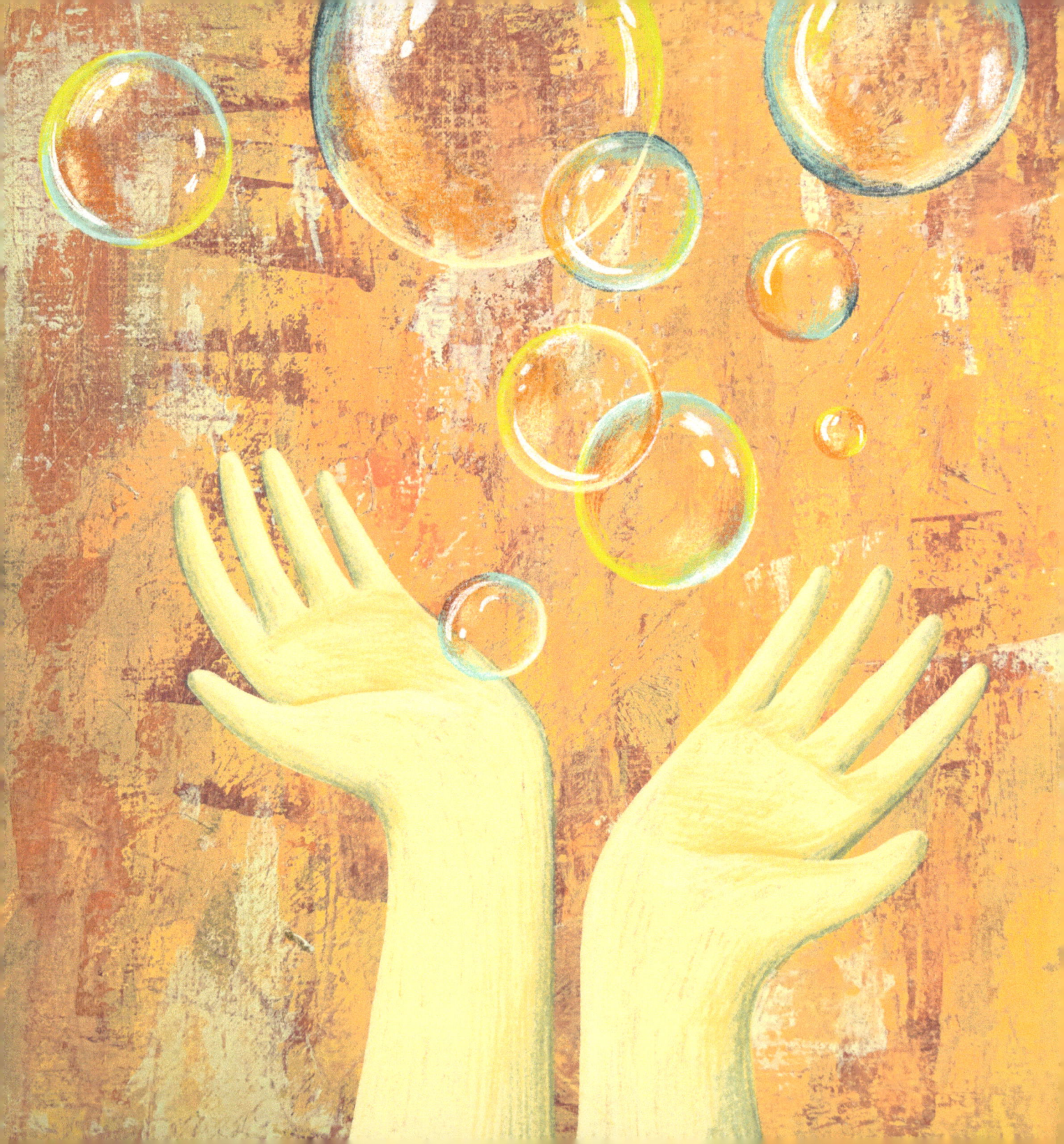

IT'S SIMPLY BLOWING BUBBLES
TO FIND CALM WITHIN
AND LET GO OF ANY STRUGGLE.
IF YOU'RE WILLING, LET'S BEGIN.

IMAGINE YOUR THOUGHTS
STRUNG UPON THE WAND.

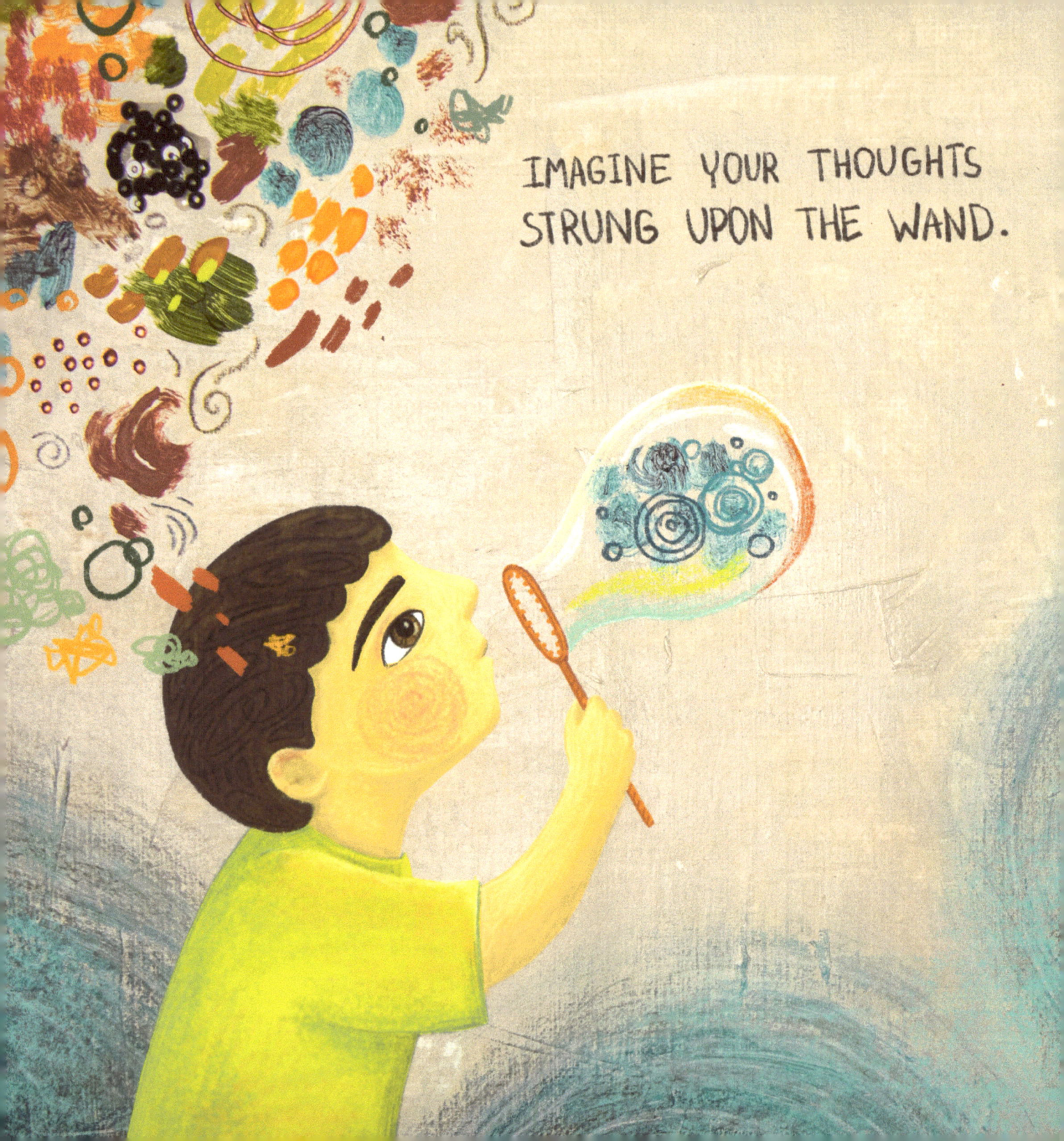

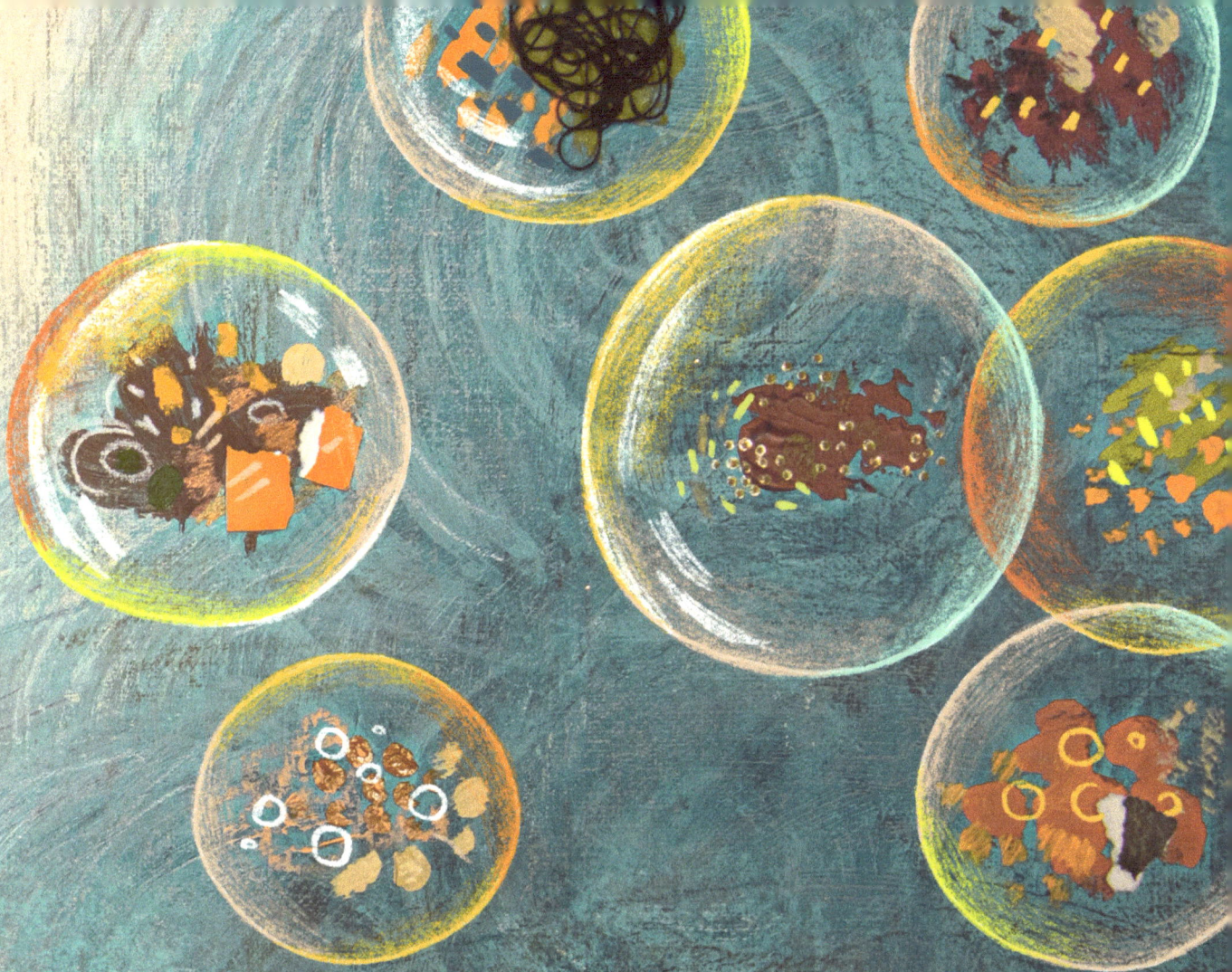

NOW FOCUS YOUR BREATH
AND SEND THEM BEYOND.

WATCH AS THEY DANCE
AND DRIFT AWAY...

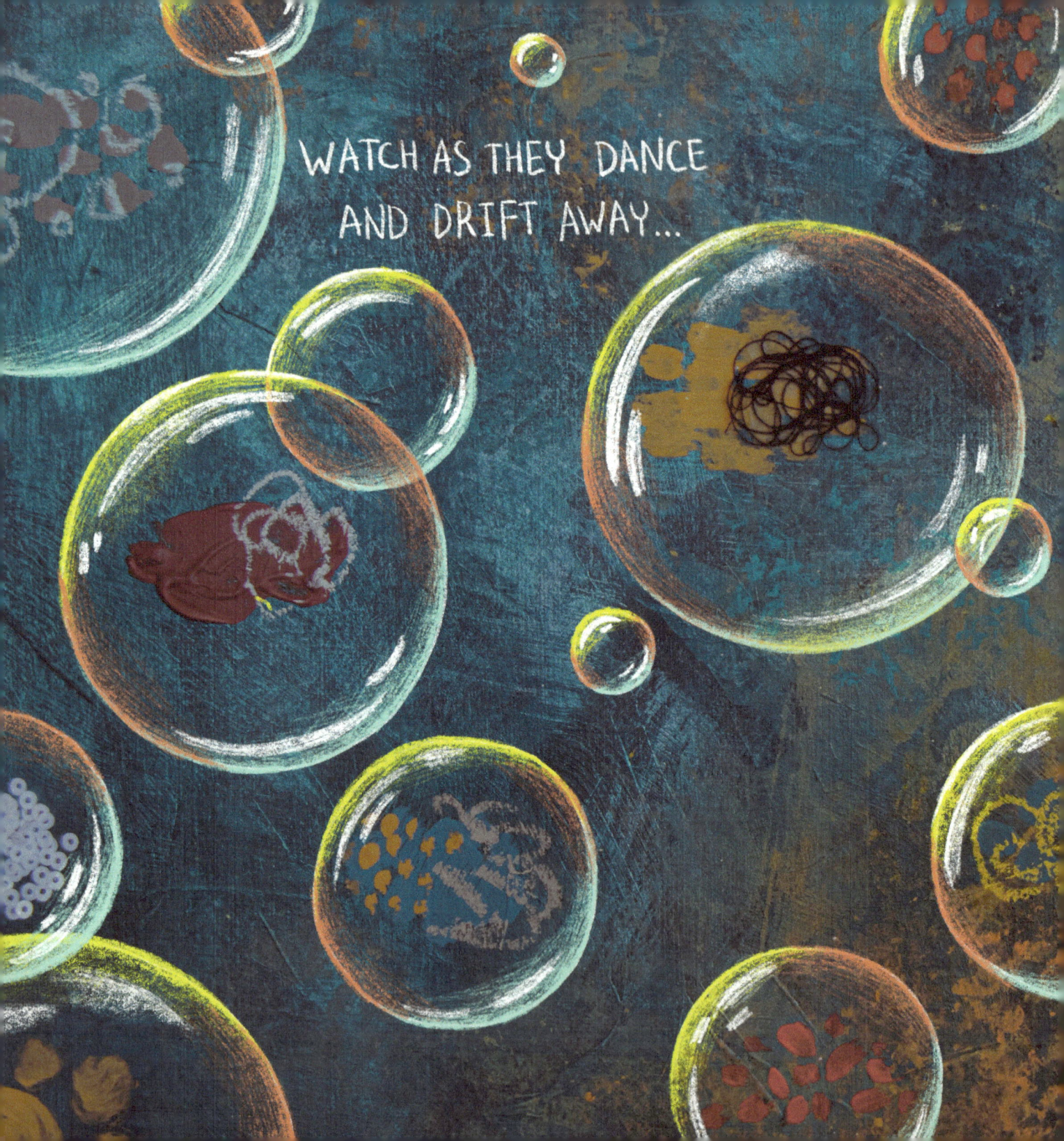

TAKE A MOMENT TO BREATHE.

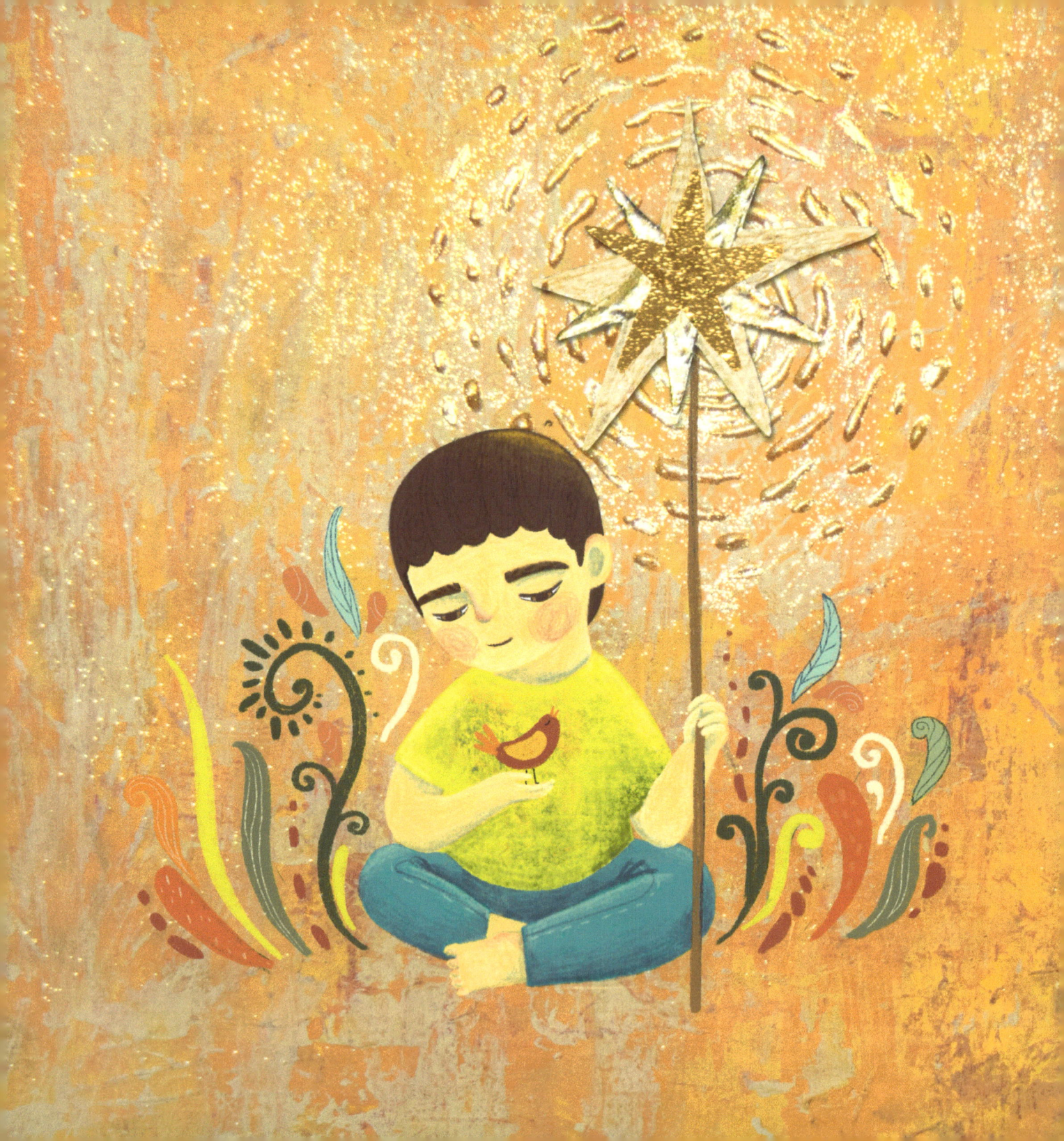

DOES YOUR MIND

FEEL CLEARER TODAY?

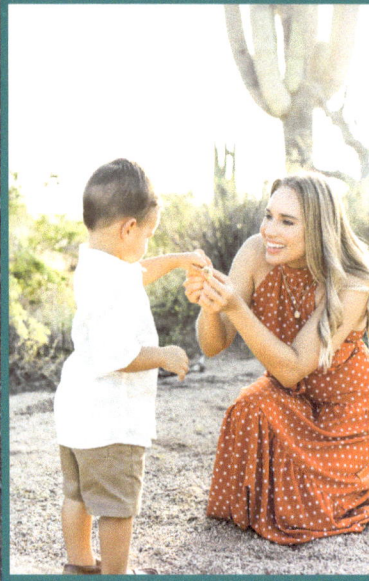

Saskia Soliz has spent the last decade supporting children with unique needs. In guiding young children, she believes in the importance of creating a nurturing environment, empowering minds, and being intentional. Her work is inspired by the six core therapeutic processes of acceptance and commitment therapy (ACT). Saskia earned her master's in curriculum and instruction with a concentration in applied behavior analysis from Arizona State University. She currently resides in Arizona with her family and enjoys the moments with her son where they are learning together through books.

To learn more about the author and her work, visit www.pinpointskillslab.com

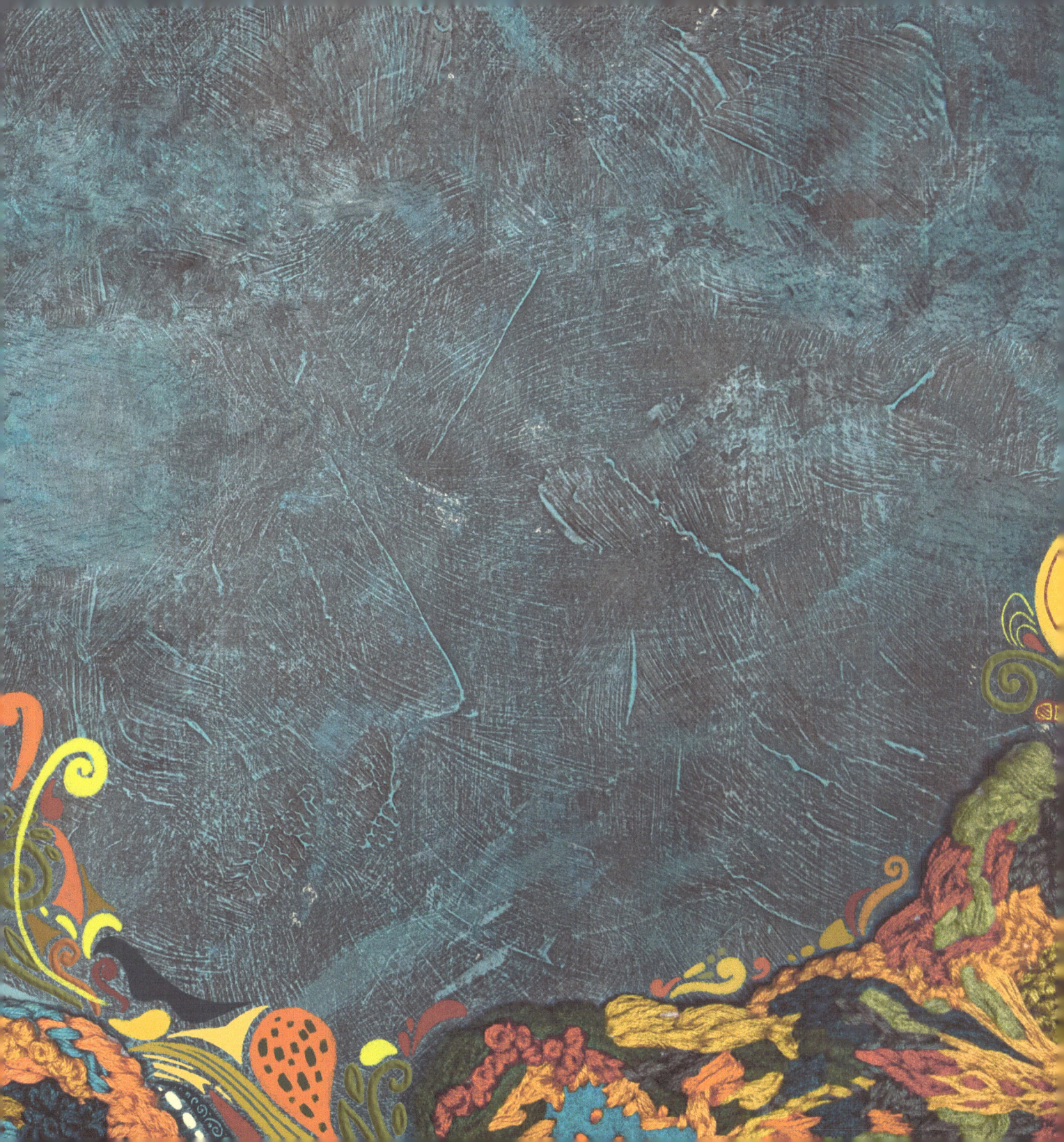

www.ingramcontent.com/pod-product-compliance
Lightning Source LLC
Chambersburg PA
CBHW061150030426
42335CB00003B/169

Every now and again, we can all use a reminder to get out of our heads and into the present moment.

ISBN 979-8-218-11919-5

9 798218 119195

IT WAS TIME

Written by Pamela Robbins

Illustrated by Eduardo Paj